Light finds its way to even the darkest of days

From Heartbeat to Heartbreak

STILLBIRTH EXPOSED

CAROLINE R POOLE

Copyright © 2018 Caroline R Poole
The moral right of the author has been asserted.

Apart from any fair dealing for the purposes of research or private study, or criticism or review, as permitted under the Copyright, Designs and Patents Act 1988, this publication may only be reproduced, stored or transmitted, in any form or by any means, with the prior permission in writing of the publishers, or in the case of reprographic reproduction in accordance with the terms of licences issued by the Copyright Licensing Agency. Enquiries concerning reproduction outside those terms should be sent to the publishers.

Matador
9 Priory Business Park,
Wistow Road, Kibworth Beauchamp,
Leicestershire. LE8 0RX
Tel: 0116 279 2299
Email: books@troubador.co.uk
Web: www.troubador.co.uk/matador
Twitter: @matadorbooks

ISBN 978 1789013 719

British Library Cataloguing in Publication Data.
A catalogue record for this book is available from the British Library.

Printed and bound by CPI Group (UK) Ltd, Croydon, CR0 4YY
Typeset in Minion Pro 11pt by Troubador Publishing Ltd, Leicester, UK

Matador is an imprint of Troubador Publishing Ltd

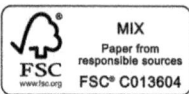

This book is dedicated to my baby girl, Olivia Ashley. Although you're not here, you're never far away. In my memories and thoughts, forever you will stay.

Always a twinkle in my sky. Love you always, Mummy.

I also dedicate this book to all of the babies gone too soon, and to every parent and their families who have had to face or are facing the difficult journey of stillbirth.

Contents

Foreword	ix
The Day I Had to Let You Go	xi
Introduction	1
Information on pre-eclampsia and HELLP syndrome	4
Secret Journey	7
The evolutionary progression of stillbirth	8
Personal story	10
What's in a heartbeat?	12
Olivia's funeral	26
Through the Storm	30
Life following stillbirth	32
Battle of the Heart	38
Number Thirteen	39
The Journey of a Teardrop	40
Rainbow of Hope	41
References	43
Acknowledgements	45

Foreword

Stillbirth has always been an emotive issue, as maternity care is an area of healthcare more commonly associated with happy outcomes. Today's midwives, particularly those without a nursing background, may find the emotional labour of caring for families experiencing pregnancy loss very difficult. The requirement for ensuring that all service users receive compassionate care (Cummings and Bennett, 2012) makes it crucial for midwives to understand stillbirth. Midwives must be able to provide compassionate, evidence-based care to women and families buffeted by the emotional storms inherent in their experience of stillbirth. Improving professionals' understanding about what parents endure when death happens at birth can positively influence the delivery of good bereavement care as the effects of poor care are far reaching (Redshaw et al., 2014). Never was this more evident than when I read Caroline's description of seeing her daughter being presented as an object; "I asked to see Olivia; just like the numerous other times during my time there… I noticed that Olivia was covered with a blanket. This was the first and only time I felt that she had been itemised. A body."

And while I feel deeply saddened by this, I truly believe that we can all learn from this account and avoid complacency, for what matters is the 'way' we approach our bereaved mothers and 'how' we do things for their families. I have spent hours listening to bereaved mothers and some have told me that the people who they thought would be there for them during this difficult time sometimes became more distant. In addition to this Caroline has so eloquently described how isolating this unique grief is and how invisible their motherhood became: "The people I know moved your existence to Mars". The woman-midwife relationship is often brief and the way midwives deliver care impacts on both. Downe et al. (2013) suggest we have "one chance to get it right". Therefore, the midwife's role is fundamental in reducing the traumatic effect of stillbirth. Training, support and enhanced communication skills have been identified as important. Otherwise, misunderstanding, miscommunication and detachment occurs, which is detrimental to providing effective and compassionate care. Gratitude is expressed to Caroline for taking this very brave step in sharing her intimate story with others. In doing so, she is raising awareness about pre-eclampsia and breaking through the barriers and secrecy that still surround the subject of stillbirth. This can only help to improve all of our understanding around such a difficult and unimaginable loss.

Mrs Christine Navin MSc., R.G.N., R.M., Adv. Dip, Couns.
Specialist Bereavement Midwife
North West L.S.A Supervisor of Midwives

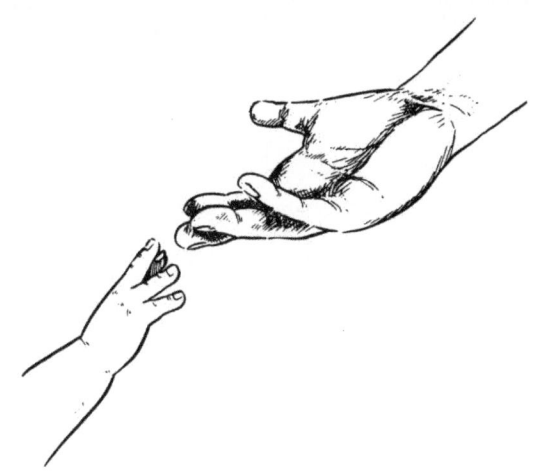

The Day I Had to Let You Go

Sitting here alone with the breeze brushing past my face,
Lost in all my thoughts, my heart rate picking up in pace.
Was this the path I chose? Or just a funny twist of fate?
A road I'm now familiar with, ever since that awful date.
My journey may have changed me, my world turned upside down,
I didn't have a choice, or even chance to smile or frown.
I didn't want to lose you, your presence was so brief,
No one ever warned me, that destiny was a thief.
Although you weren't here long, nothing can take away,
My memories, thoughts and feelings, they are here to stay.
My heart still yearns to see you, the pain will never go,
I will always love you, more than anyone will know.
All the things I will never know, like the colour of your eyes,
Then there's all the things you miss, from sunset to sunrise.
Maybe I was supposed to learn the things that I now know,
But my life changed forever on the day I had to let you go.

By the age of twenty it is hard to know much about not only life, but about yourself as an individual; to know what path to take and which people in your life are the most important; who will be there for you in times where it matters, and who will disappear during your darkest hours. Not only are you learning your own boundaries as a human being, you are continuously being perceived as an individual by a society full of stereotypes, trying to mould you into believing things that people tell you about yourself which could be far from the truth. There are certain circumstances in which society can be either very accepting or disapproving, and it has been my experience that to be pregnant at a young age these days puts you nearer to that disapproving category. I'm talking from my own experience as, at the age of twenty, I was pregnant and just as clueless about pregnancy as anybody embarking on their first pregnancy would be, regardless of their age or circumstances. Every individual has a different experience and story to tell. If each of us were open to different views or situations, it would be nice to think that instead of judging people by stereotypes or shutting off in fear that somebody would not like what we were saying, we could find that actually we might want to talk about the things that society labels as "unacceptable". We might learn that it is society alone that denies us from being taken as an individual and dictates which subjects in our lives are inappropriate to talk about.

There are many individual circumstances deemed as "unacceptable" to society. Many of these situations are experienced by a high number of people from all walks of life. People who would never cross paths, but are bound by the same misconception of society regarding their circumstance. Similarities in people who have so much in common but society dictates them to be so far apart.

I have already mentioned the negative outlook of society regarding pregnancy at a young age, but my experience has also taught me that, although society may be quick to judge certain circumstances, filtering people into categories based on a certain aspect of their life, there are circumstances from which society is quick to shy away, and it is these circumstances that are labelled as "unacceptable".

If we can be judged and categorised so easily in so many different aspects of our lives, then why is it that some of the most important parts of our lives can be avoided and ignored? "Unacceptable" to talk about, deprived of any knowledge and not allowed to be understood. All of the petty things used to scrutinise us, yet when we could do with a bit of guidance or someone to talk to, we suddenly find ourselves isolated by society and unable to allow our thoughts and feelings any recognition. It is only during our most challenging times that society lets go of our hand and leaves us to find our own way through the dark, hoping that ignorance will somehow override our need to acknowledge something in which society alone doesn't consider to be plausible.

There are so many of these circumstances that as a society we continue to deny. What we fail to realise is that if we stopped to think about all of the individuals who are each walking their own lonely path, if we could somehow build bridges to allow one another access onto our own individual path, we may provide ourselves with answers to the questions that we don't dare to ask. Could we find comfort in our loneliness and realise that whatever we are dealing with isn't actually as alien as society allows it to be?

The reason I am comparing the ways in which we are categorised and judged by society based on certain aspects of our lives, and the "unacceptable" subjects that are avoided by society, is that when I became pregnant at twenty, I found myself dealing with both of the above. Going from being categorised by an opinionated society to my circumstance being completely avoided and written off, when twenty-six weeks and two days into my pregnancy my baby girl was stillborn after I developed severe pre-eclampsia and HELLP syndrome.

I was previously unaware of these pregnancy-related illnesses, so I would like to share the following information to help raise awareness of these potentially life-threatening conditions:

Pre-eclampsia is potentially a very dangerous condition associated only with pregnancy. Pre-eclampsia is new hypertension, generally presenting after twenty weeks or shortly after delivery, with significant proteinuria (protein in the urine). Severe pre-eclampsia is pre-eclampsia with severe hypertension and/or with symptoms and/or biochemical and/or haematological impairment. Eclampsia is a convulsive condition associated with pre-eclampsia.

Pre-eclampsia can sometimes present symptomless or resemble "normal" effects of pregnancy, which is why all antenatal appointments are vital. Symptoms of pre-eclampsia may include one or more of the following:

- Severe headache
- Vision problems (such as blurred vision, spots/flashing lights)
- Sudden swelling of the face, hands or feet (oedema)
- Pain below the ribs or vomiting (not morning sickness)
- Reduced baby movement

There are a number of factors that can increase the risk of developing pre-eclampsia, such as:

- First pregnancy
- If you had pre-eclampsia during a previous pregnancy
- Family history of pre-eclampsia (e.g. your mother or sister has had pre-eclampsia)
- Multiple pregnancy (e.g. twins or triplets)
- Pregnancy interval of more than ten years
- If you are over the age of forty
- If you have a body mass index (BMI) of thirty or more at your first visit

The exact cause of pre-eclampsia is not known, although it is thought to occur due to a problem with the placenta. One theory suggested by the NHS Choices webpage is that the problems are due to the development of the blood vessels to the placenta during the early stages of pregnancy. Whilst the blood vessels in the womb are supposed to change shape and become wider, feeding the villi nutrients (root-like growths produced by a fertilised egg, which anchor it to the lining of the womb), it is a theory that, in the case of pre-eclampsia, these blood vessels do not fully transform, causing poor blood supply through the placenta to the baby. Unborn babies of women with pre-eclampsia tend to have slow growth due to receiving less oxygen and nutrients which is known as intra-uterine or foetal growth restriction. The only cure for pre-eclampsia is for both the baby and the placenta to be delivered.

HELLP syndrome is a serious complication of pregnancy in which there is a combined liver and blood clotting disorder. HELLP stands for the following:

- H – Haemolysis (rupture of the red blood cells)
- EL – Elevated Liver (enzymes in the blood)
- LP – Low Platelet count

There is an ongoing debate on whether HELLP syndrome is a severe form of pre-eclampsia or a separate condition altogether, as it may be preceded by clear signs of pre-eclampsia, but can also arise out of the blue without any of the classic warning signs. The typical presenting symptom of HELLP syndrome is pain below the ribs which is sometimes accompanied by vomiting and headaches. Often confused with heartburn, the pain is often very severe and is associated with tenderness of the liver.

HELLP syndrome is a maternal problem and may be associated with one or more of the following problems:

- Severely disturbed blood clotting function, leading to heavy uncontrollable bleeding, particularly after surgery.
- Severe liver damage, which can lead to failure or even rupture of this vital organ.
- Severe kidney problems, including kidney failure.
- Breathing difficulties (which may be severe enough for the mother to need artificial ventilation)
- Stroke

HELLP syndrome is a life-threatening condition in which the only cure is delivery of the baby and placenta.

Secret Journey

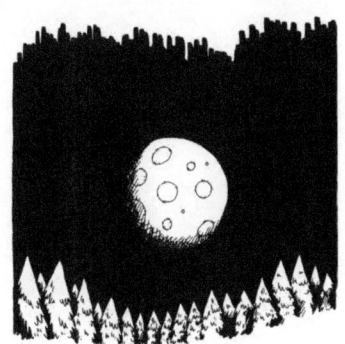

As my eyes open, I face a new day,
The hurt I can feel always finds its way,
The battle I'm fighting is one I can't win,
Emotions and feelings so hard to sink in.
How did this happen? Why did you go?
I can't be complete, but no-one will know,
Plunged into the unknown, in this unspoken deal,
Where it seems I can't talk about you, how is this real?
Often I'm voiceless, trapped in a lie,
But inside it breaks me, as I ask myself why?
The nights seem so dark, eerie and long,
I remember what happened, why is this wrong?
The moon seems lost, up in the stars,
The people I know moved your existence to Mars.
Out of this world, reality a sham,
Everything in question, all that I am.
The Earth carried on spinning, the sun chose to rise,
The warmth of its presence drying my eyes,
As life carries on, it's like no-one can see,
The pain of my journey, travelled only by me.
The colours of the sky will always remain,
But my life as I knew it will never be the same.

In the U.K, around fifteen babies a day are stillborn, or die within the first twenty-eight days of life. As a society, we have evolved in many ways regarding our approach to stillbirth. Not too long ago, stillborn babies were disposed of as if they had never existed. The families of these babies weren't able to see or hold their baby and were expected to carry on as before, despite having to live with the heartache that comes with losing a child.

Thankfully, these days, families are encouraged to spend time with their baby and are able to have photographs, as well as hand and footprints amongst other keepsakes, allowing them to make memories and grieve for their baby. By law in England and Wales, babies that are stillborn after twenty-four weeks gestation have to have their birth and death registered, allowing them official recognition and the right to a funeral.

Although this is a big step forward, I still feel that in many other ways stillbirth is generally a prohibited subject to society. The expectation to carry on as before still lingers, expressions such as "you will get over it" or "you can try again" seem to be acceptable comments to make regarding the death of a baby, but if your grandma died, would you just "get over it" or want another one? Would you choose to forget about her or never want to talk about her again? If somebody mentioned her name, or spoke about the things she said or did, reminding you of times you shared with her, would your grief become that unbearable that you would be unable to cope? If you avoided speaking about her, would this mean that you would forget she existed at all? If you had the option to forget her very existence, would you want to do so because living with her memory is far too distressing and painful? The truth is that regardless of how long a loved one is with us, nobody would want to forget about them, or choose to think of them as an illusion, acting as though they never existed.

As a society, if we are able to keep an open mind about the death of a grandparent, or someone who has lived long enough for acceptable recognition, then I feel that we should be able to extend our minds to dealing with the death of a baby. Choosing to be blind to something that happens every day doesn't change the fact that it happens. Whether this is acceptable to society or not, the reality is that however any of us deal with anything remains the same irrespective of us talking about it or not.

Before I share my personal experience that I live with every day, I would like to say that my baby girl, Olivia, is always in my thoughts and will always have a special place in my heart. Although the time we had together was so short, she has touched my life in more ways than I could have ever imagined. Through every anniversary and the milestones I will never see her reach, I will always be grateful for the time that we had and I am proud to be her mummy. I love you Olivia.

From the moment I found out I was pregnant in November 2009, my feelings and the journey that followed are still very clear in my mind. From the initial shock, to the excitement and the slight fear of the unknown, there was no doubt in my mind that I wanted the best for my baby. I enjoyed reading every baby book I could get my hands on and loved keeping track of my baby's development. From the excitement of my first scan, to magical moments such as hearing my baby's heartbeat for the first time and feeling my baby move. My due date was confirmed for the Twenty-fifth of July 2010, and my twenty-two week scan revealed I was having a little girl. Apart from being small for her gestation, in which I was reassured and booked in for another ultrasound in a further four weeks' time, my pregnancy was progressing as it should have been.

On the morning of Monday 19th April, I was getting ready for work when for a second or two I felt disorientated, resulting in me losing my balance and stumbling as a wave of dizziness came over me. Looking back, I feel like this was a funny turn; perhaps an indication that something was wrong, or a sign to warn me of what was to come. I quickly returned to normal and, due to this being my first pregnancy and not knowing what was, in fact, normal or not, as well as my follow-up scan now a matter of days away, I made the decision to carry on my day as planned, which still to this day fills me with regret.

As early evening approached, a sharp pain developed around my shoulder blade. I recalled a conversation I had earlier in the day with a work colleague who complained of backache. I remember thinking that it must have been something similar to what he had been describing, so was initially quite dismissive. The pain, however, was constant and like nothing I had ever felt before. I thought a hot bath would help, convincing myself that I had pulled a muscle, but my attempts to stop the pain were of no avail.

The pain continued to intensify, becoming unbearable. After crawling around on the floor in agony and numerous failed attempts to sleep the pain off, I started to worry that something was wrong. I didn't like the idea of taking painkillers as I worried how they would affect my baby. With the pain starting in my chest, as well as it getting late into the night, I decided to ring the NHS helpline for some reassurance on taking some paracetamol. I thought I would sound daft, but my only concern at this point was for my baby to be all right. The conversation that followed resulted in an ambulance being sent and I was rushed to hospital.

On admission to A & E, despite the pain I was in, I wondered why I was there. Although I thought it would be a matter of discussing what painkillers I could take before being discharged, I felt comforted that I would be checked over before leaving. Making sure that whatever pain relief I would be prescribed would be all right to take and that my baby would be safe. My blood pressure was checked and at 200/101, although it seemed very high compared to my 110/64 observed by my midwife only three days before, I felt reassured that it had dropped slightly from when the paramedics had checked it before my admission to hospital. Routine tests also revealed that I had a very high level of protein in my urine and I was told that I needed to be transferred to the delivery suite. I thought it seemed odd, but put it down to routine because I was pregnant. Slightly confused and starting to worry again, I remained calm, distracting my thoughts by rationalising how tired I would feel getting up for work in the morning, but as I got to the delivery suite the scene that unfolded will be etched into my memory forever…

What's in a heartbeat?

That strong, steady sound,
Something during pregnancy which is normally found.
I remember the first time that I heard your heart beat,
My precious baby girl, whom I was longing to meet.
As weeks went by, my bump started to show,
I felt you move as you continued to grow,
What was to come? If only I knew,
I took you for granted, I hadn't a clue.
What happened next, I wasn't prepared,
I didn't know what was happening, but I knew I was scared.
Rushed into hospital during the night,

Back pain and chest pain, nothing felt right.
Pre-eclampsia and HELLP, nothing made sense,
Everything seemed serious, the doctors seemed tense.
Everything surreal, what did it mean?
To answer my questions, no-one seemed keen.
What about my baby? Tell me she's safe,
Waiting for the ultrasound, I had to keep faith.
What's in a heartbeat? My whole life it seems,
My trust and my fate, my hopes and my dreams.
The doctor was quiet, something was wrong,
Another came over, the seconds seemed long.
I asked for an answer, I needed to know,
Somebody tell me, my tears ready to flow.
"I'm sorry there's no heartbeat," those were his words,
My world crashed down, such words seemed absurd.
I couldn't take it in, how could this be?
Nothing made sense, at least not to me.
My baby was gone, she couldn't have died,
I knew what it meant, but what if they lied?
Another scan confirmed this nightmare was true,
How could all this come out of the blue?
What's in a heartbeat? One that's now still?
Loneliness and emptiness that nothing can fill.
Eventually I was induced and my baby was born,
My world fell apart and my emotions were torn.
From the second I saw her, until I last kissed her cheek,
Goodbye seemed so final, my insides turned weak.
Longing for one more hold of her hand,
My arms reached out lost in a faraway land.
What's in a heartbeat? A flicker of hope,

Memories and love which help me to cope.
Sadness and guilt, this may be true,
But as long as my heart beats, I will always love you.

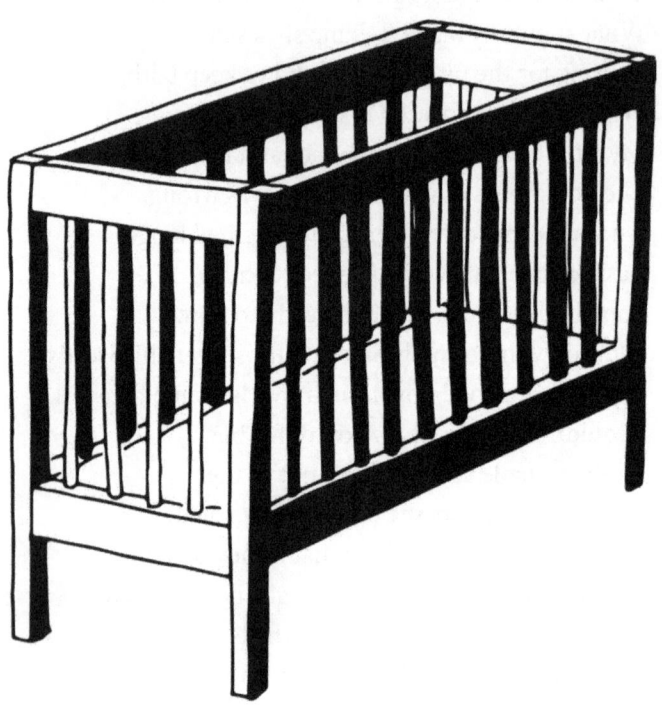

Going from making that initial phone call to having to digest the seriousness of my condition was so surreal I felt as though I had arrived on the set of casualty. Being greeted by more doctors than I had ever seen in my life and learning that I was at risk of going into a coma, having a seizure, heart attack or stroke at any minute was not only scary, but seemed so absurd I thought that my notes must have been mixed up with someone else's and that they were going to kill me. The reality was that I had severe pre-eclampsia and HELLP syndrome. My organs were shutting down and I had swelling around my brain. My body was retaining fluid causing the onset of oedema and as my blood pressure fluctuated it remained persistently high. Whilst critically ill, I went on to learn that my baby girl had died due to the complications of pre-eclampsia and HELLP. After making no sense of this at first, a second ultrasound was arranged from which the eerie image I was presented with will always be with me. Normally my little girl was very active during an ultrasound scan, but this time everything was still. There was no sign of a heartbeat and as I looked at her lying motionless at the bottom of the screen, so peaceful and still, the reality that there really was no heartbeat crept upon me, shattering my heart into pieces. My baby had died.

After the longest night of my life, my blood pressure, although still dangerously high, had dropped enough to allow me to be induced. I was told that the only cure for my condition was for the baby and the placenta to be delivered, but that was a decision I felt was made a lot quicker than I had anticipated. I was still clinging on to some hope that the doctors could be wrong, and I didn't feel ready to face up to the reality that I would have to give birth to a baby that wouldn't be alive. My labour progressed slowly and I was induced a total of three times that day. Throughout the contractions and the pain I was still suffering with my back, the thought that my baby may have had a faint heartbeat which had been overlooked because she was poorly too made the prospect of delivery that little less scary.

My labour eventually came to an end. At 20:56 on Tuesday 20th April my little girl was born silently into the world. Everything I thought the birth of my baby would be was gone. The room filled with sadness and instead of the sound of a baby's first cry, an eerie silence and the feeling of hopelessness took its place.

It seemed like a long time before anybody spoke. Throughout my pregnancy I had wondered what my little girl would look like. I wondered what colour her hair would be and about the colour of her eyes. When I was first told that she would be stillborn I remember recalling information that I had retained from history lessons at school. I associated stillbirth with something that Henry VIII wives had suffered, and had no other knowledge or reason to believe that it affected people or even happened in this day and age. Nothing could have prepared me for what was now a living nightmare that I couldn't wake up from. I knew before I was asked that I wanted to meet my little girl, but as she was prepared for me to see I felt apprehensive about what to expect.

As I laid eyes on my newborn daughter for the first time, my fears and anxiety instantly disappeared. She was wrapped and lay peacefully in the foetal position within a wicker basket. My hand automatically reached out to touch her. She was warm and her skin felt so soft. As I stroked her little face my hand shook a little. She was so perfectly formed, with a little button nose and long fingers and feet. The first thing she wore was a hand knitted white dress, which had a mostly pink and purple dotted pattern, hinted with a touch of pale green at the top. It tied at the front with a soft pink ribbon and looked delicate yet pretty. I held her tiny hand between my fingers and some time passed before she was taken to be weighed and measured.

Starting the physical recovery from pre-eclampsia and HELLP syndrome meant a longer stay in hospital, which saw my transfer from high dependency back to a room on a delivery suite and then finally to the bereavement suite. I still remember the first time I was able to have a shower after my admission. It shocked me how weak my body was when I stood up for the first time. I felt dizzy and faint, but in my mind I was determined to walk what must have been five to ten steps and shower myself, despite having to be watched by a member of staff. Although I had a longer stay in hospital than I originally expected, I got to spend a lot of time with my little girl, which I will treasure forever. I thought about names a lot whilst I was pregnant, especially after I found out that I was expecting a baby girl. The name I kept going back to and thinking over was Olivia Ashley. I thought it sounded pretty so I felt this would be the most fitting name for my little girl.

Within the time that I spent with Olivia, I spent a lot of it having cuddles with her. She lay in bed with me and I would tell her things about the world, and about the things that I had planned for us to do. I cried telling her how much I loved her and apologised because I felt that I had let her down. Sometimes I wondered why I hadn't died instead, feeling guilty that I had survived our ordeal. Other times the realisation of how lucky I was to get to hospital when I did was haunting, and the constant reminder of how suddenly everything changed absolutely terrified me.

Not long after Olivia's birth, one of the midwives gave me two tablets that would stop my breast milk. She explained to me that although Olivia had died, my body would only register that I had given birth and would continue to function as if I'd had a live birth. I looked at the tablets as she walked away. A wave of sadness came over me as I thought about what she had said. I understood that it made sense to take them, but I couldn't bring myself to do it. I had lost my baby and felt upset by the thought of losing something else connected to her existence before I had to. I felt guilty hiding them, but at the time it felt like the only thing I could do until I was able to dispose of them.

On Thursday 22nd April, Olivia had a naming and blessing service. Her birth and death were registered formally on Tuesday 27th April. Although she didn't have a post-mortem, her cause of death was registered as pre-eclampsia. Intra-uterine death and prematurity were also listed on her certificate as evidence of her stillbirth. Olivia did have an external medical examination in which no external abnormalities were found.

Throughout my time at the hospital, the staff were amazing. Without their care, I honestly don't know where I would be today. The care that both Olivia and I received was beyond words; always attentive, friendly and warm, as well as patient with all of my questions. I still feel that the care we were given went far beyond any job description. Olivia was always well cared for by all of the staff at the hospital and treated just like any other newborn baby. It saddens me to go on to this, but towards the end of my hospital stay, I asked to see Olivia; just like the numerous other times during my time there. It was getting late and the lady I had asked wasn't a member of staff that I had seen before. She didn't seem as friendly as the midwives I was used to, but did say she would bring Olivia to me. Some time passed before she reappeared, but as she came through the door I noticed that Olivia was covered with a blanket. I was mortified as she awkwardly placed the Moses basket on the bed and left the room without saying a word. As I got to the bed from where I was sitting, I felt sad as the reality of death hit me once again. I quickly reached out to pull the white cover back as I couldn't stand the thought of Olivia lying underneath it like an object, or the typical image you think of in relation to "a body". That body was my daughter and as I pulled the cover back expecting to see my baby carefully dressed in the normal cared-for manner I was used to, my stomach churned as I found two body identification labels taped on top of her. This was the first and only time I felt that she had been itemised. A body. Identified by a name on a piece of paper, dismissing any human relation or emotions, with the only significance of being part of a sad and lonely process. I quickly pulled the labels off her and lifted her out of the Moses basket. I sat for a minute and then picked the labels up, glancing again at the information in front of me. They looked exactly as you would expect. A simple yet formal layout with a bold, black border and a very morbid appearance. This was bad enough, but it upset me to see Olivia's name written on these labels to certify the identification of her "body". It also traumatised me to see my own name written above tick boxes for burial or cremation in reference to funeral arrangements, whilst still recovering from being very ill myself. I didn't see the lady who brought Olivia to me that night again.

Shortly after that experience, my own hospital admission started drawing to an end. The day before I was discharged, Olivia had to be transferred to the main mortuary of the hospital. I went with her, and spent some time with her in the chapel of rest because I didn't want her to have to go on her own. I also knew that this would be the last night that we would both be at the hospital, so I wanted to try and find the words to say goodbye. That night I found it difficult to sleep. My heart broke as I looked at her photographs, knowing that she was at the other side of the hospital lying in the mortuary. I felt lost as it dawned on me that I would have to leave the hospital without her.

As the next day came around, the inevitable task of going home without Olivia was upon me. I will never forget the feeling of emptiness that consumed me as I walked out to see a couple gently placing their newborn baby into their car; my stomach churned trying to digest the sea of pink in this ironic twist of fate. I had gone into hospital pregnant, with my hopes and future plans intact, but as I stopped to take one last look at the hospital, my heart and arms physically ached for my baby. Against every instinct within me, I turned to walk away, causing loneliness and grief to surge once again through my entire body. I left with photographs amongst my bags, taking bittersweet memories but having to leave my baby girl behind.

I spent the couple of weeks that followed visiting Olivia at the hospital. I hadn't been to a funeral before, but within this time I was faced with having to make the uneasy decision of how my little girl would be laid to rest. It would have been a lonely few weeks without the reassurance and guidance of the funeral director, for which I will always be grateful. There was always a lot of pink around Olivia, so I decided that it should be a significant colour at her funeral. I had grown up enjoying Disney films, and whilst I was pregnant I had looked forward to the day where I could snuggle up on the sofa with Olivia and watch them again. For this reason, I chose the song "Can you feel the love tonight" by Elton John as the first song for her funeral.

With the arrangements for Olivia's funeral coming together, I wanted to do all that I could for her. I decided to write her a letter that she would be buried with. This is my own copy of Olivia's letter, which has always remained something between Olivia and myself until now. Although there are parts of it that I find difficult to read now as I look back, I feel that it does expose some of my thoughts during this time.

To my beautiful baby girl,

Hope you're okay, sweetie. Mummy misses you so much. I want you to know that I am so proud to be your mummy and feel very lucky to have such a special little girl. You are so perfect and beautiful in every way; everything about you is so gorgeous and cute. I feel blessed to have you in my life, although our time together here has been so short. Thank you for showing me the true meaning of love and for opening my eyes to the cruelty of life. One day there will be answers and I hope that Mummy can do some good things that will help other people. I wish so much we could have stayed together, but you were too good for this world. The angels only call the best people before they reach all of the cruelty and nasty things in this world; so have fun playing with those angels and know that you have only taken a step in front of me. One day we will be together again, and when we are we will never part again. Mummy and Daddy, and all of your grandmas, grandads, aunties and uncles, are still doing nice things for you. We all love and miss you and we will forever remember the precious times that we did share here. Thank you for touching our lives. You hold a special place in our hearts, and always will do. Remember that you are only a thought away, and you can come back to me in my dreams until that day comes when we can finally be together again.

Sleep tight, little princess, until the day we meet again. I love you so much.

Mummy

Xxxxxxxx

The day before her funeral, Olivia was transferred to the funeral home from the hospital. I felt anxious that day and, although I had agreed not to go, I couldn't sit back without knowing that she would be all right there. I was supposed to have said my final goodbyes to Olivia earlier that week at the hospital. It felt strange that I hadn't seen her when I knew I would never have that option again once her funeral had been. I needed to see my baby one last time. I spoke to the funeral director and decided I would spend that last moment with my little girl and say one last goodbye.

Just after I got to the funeral home, the private ambulance that had been to pick Olivia up from the hospital arrived. I felt numb as I watched it pull in. I had to wait a little while before I was able to go into the chapel of rest to see her. I had chosen a baby pink colour for her coffin, which was lined with pink silk. The finality of death hung over me once again as I walked into the room to see Olivia laying in her coffin. The room itself was neutral in colour and had a reassuring, peaceful feel to it. I stayed with Olivia for a while, holding her little hand between my fingers one last time. She was wrapped in a blanket and wore a white rabbit hat and pink stripy socks that had her name on over her little pink and white bunny baby grow. I traced my fingers over the silver pendant of the necklace I was wearing as I looked at the matching one Olivia wore. I thought that it would give us another connection when I could no longer see her if we had special necklaces that matched. I felt sad knowing that I would never see her again once I left, but told her that she would always be with me and I was going to miss her because I loved her so much. Along with her letter and little teddy, which wore a butterfly tag with her name on, she had another little heart pendant which I placed over her heart. The funeral director came into the room just before I left. After asking him a final few questions about Olivia's funeral, he told me that the lid would be placed on her coffin after I had left. He then asked me if I would like to be the last person to see Olivia and do that job. It remains one of the hardest things I have done in my life. I kissed my baby girl on the forehead and whispered my final words to her, before placing the lid onto her little coffin.

I must have been on autopilot after waking up the next morning. I felt a mixture of emotions having to get ready for the day that no parent should face. It was Friday 14th May, the day of my daughter's funeral…

Olivia's Funeral

A dull image is silently sketched by the sky,
Clouds start to gather, withholding their cry,
In the order of life, this is a fault,
But the hearsette arrives and comes to a halt.
Before living at all, now on one final journey,
To plead this case for my baby, I have no attorney,
As I sit down beside her, my mind starts to think,
So helpless sitting next to her tiny coffin in pink,
On the outside I'm numb, inside I cry,
Looking out of the window as the world rolls on by,
Emotions within me plead this to stop,
Whilst physically my body acts like a prop,
Time is unruly, playing a cruel and harsh game,
It gives a call for her service, disregarding her name,
Haunted by flashbacks, I'm attacked by anxiety,
Trapped in a ritual, unmapped by society.
Words echo around me, seeming afar,
Twinkle twinkle little star,
My heart is on trial, despite how I plea,
Fate locked it up and threw away the key,
As if in a courtroom amongst the judge and the jury,
All gathered to hear the final part of this story,
Warm tears fill my eyes as I try not to blink,
A lump in my throat, its timing in sync,
I stand in the witness box, struggling to speak,
The case is adjourned, the outcome is bleak.
An absence of justice, a truancy of sins,
A new scene unfolds, the committal begins,
Resisting a protest, without making a sound,

My little girl's coffin is placed in the ground.
Rose petals replace soil, so delicate and small,
Still torturing my mind whilst I'm watching them fall,
As the service concludes, and draws to an end,
The sun sneaks through the clouds and offers me a friend,
Directing its warmth, it shines with an aim,
Beaming down on the coffin, reflecting her name,
Releasing balloons up to the sky,
The sun gives a smile to this final goodbye,
Holding onto our time together, I'll always feel blessed,
As I let go of our future and lay my baby to rest.

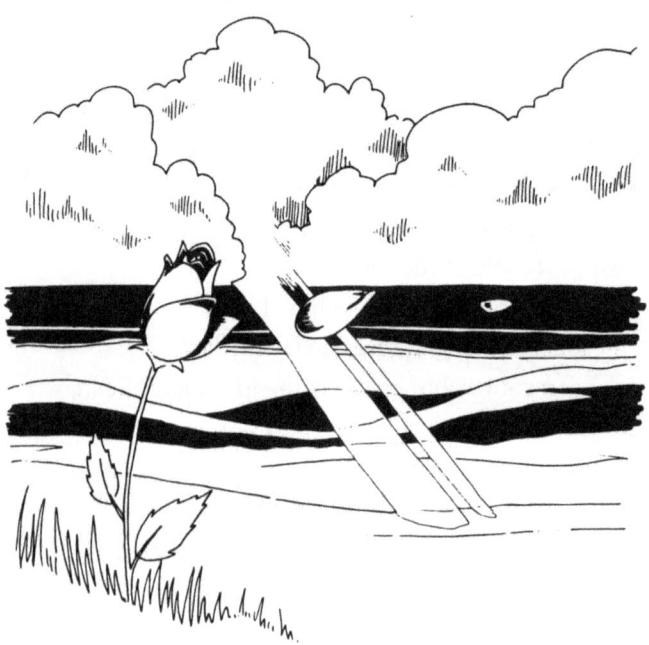

The journey I've been on since losing Olivia has taught me a lot, not only about myself, but about what is important in life; as well as reasons why nothing should be taken for granted. I have had my eyes opened to the flaws of society and have realised that regardless of whether certain circumstances are widely accepted or not, it doesn't change the situations that we as individuals may face, nor does it make our journey any less significant. If we find ourselves isolated by society during our most challenging times, it is then that we learn who is there for us and realise that it is society alone that struggles to comprehend our personal circumstances. Disregarding the often dismissive response of society when it comes to stillbirth, the failure to recognise the impact of day to day living with stillbirth doesn't mean that it will disappear. This day to day living with stillbirth is something that I like to compare to the structure of a leaf. Each leaf is unique, reflecting the differences and experiences in each individual life. Looking at a leaf as if it were mapping out your life, the main veins would be representing the main choices and paths in your life. The smaller veins which you have to look closer to see, are still important and represent different aspects of your life and each tell their own story about your experiences.

When you look at the overall structure of a leaf in this way, it highlights that when everything you go through in your life is put together, it creates your own personal story, which not only makes you unique as a person but also shows the significance each of your experiences has in your life, whether they can be overlooked or not. Going back to stillbirth, dismissing the loss of a baby to "just one of those things" or something you "get over" doesn't erase that part of your story, whether it can be overlooked by others or not. Yes, you learn to live with it, but just like the small veins on a leaf, the loss of a baby remains a part of your life and has a place on the map of your overall journey.

My perception of life and the course of my own journey certainly changed throughout my own stillbirth experience. Losing Olivia has left an impact on my life. It may not have been the one I imagined, but I remain grateful for all of the good that has followed and for the lessons that I have learned so far. I believe that positive things can be found hiding amongst our darker days, even though some of our challenges occur from realms far beyond anything we could ever anticipate. As my book draws to an end and my own experience of stillbirth goes back to an undisclosed area of my life, I would like to conclude by saying the following: As the years pass by with a continued silence instead of any mention of Olivia's name; when the very mention of her name creates an awkwardness that swallows her existence; when I'm expected to have forgotten her presence or I'm supposed to be "over it"; I would like to say that whether society can accept my personal circumstances or not, it will never change what has happened or take away the love that I will always have for Olivia. She is never far from my mind and is the inspiration behind my determination to help others through this difficult journey. Now and then when I reach out for the hand I will never be able to hold, I remember the little girl who touched my life that I will never see grow up. She may not be here now but, just like the small veins of a leaf, her presence will always be a part of my life. I may have buried my baby girl, but with her I buried the daughter I will never have.

Through the Storm

When the sea becomes rough, and there's no place to run,
There's nothing but hopelessness shadowing the sun,
So powerful and bold, it can trigger your fears,
Overwhelming in size, it doesn't notice your tears,
No sympathy is shown, it continues its rage,
It locks what you think back up in its cage,
Summoning the clouds as it swallows the shore,
The sky just as angry as it lets out a roar,
Clouds black and heavy as the thunder rolls by,
Lightning crashes as it lights up the sky,
Just when it seems it's not possible for more,
The clouds erupt and the rain starts to pour,
Lost in the storm losing faith to get out,
That's when the sky has its last shout,
Everything is calm, no danger in sight,
The sun stills the waves reflecting its light,
Not a cloud in the sky, the breeze ever so slight,
The sea now transparent, you forget all your fright,
So peaceful and welcoming now everything's blue,
No trace of a storm, or the fear you once knew,
Now everything is tranquil, the disaster is hidden,
But you will never forget the storm you have ridden.

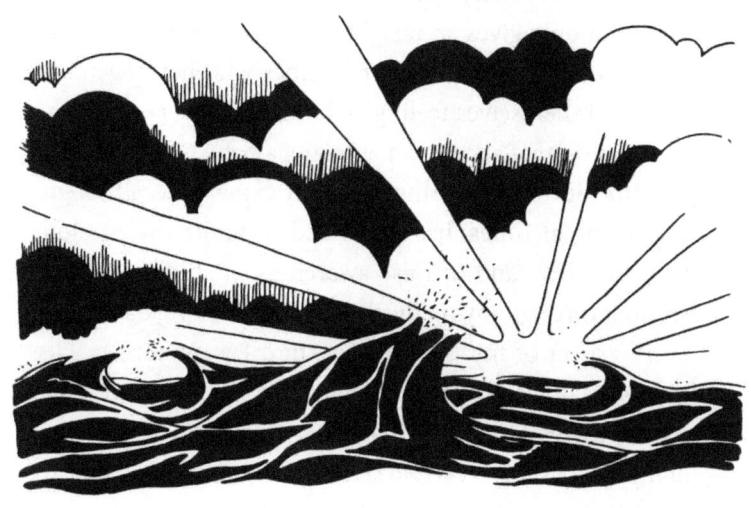

A few years have gone by now since I made the decision to relive my journey with Olivia to produce a book that I hope not only gives an insight into my stillbirth, but also holds out that hand to other families who have been, or may find themselves feeling isolated in the dark with the devastation that accompanies losing a baby.

The journey of writing about my experience, although harrowing at times, has continued to ignite my passion to help others and to raise awareness of stillbirth. After reading through my medical notes and looking back over every aspect of my personal journey, I wanted to tackle the issues of why stillbirth is still a taboo subject amongst society today, as well as tell my own story through the eyes of my then twenty-year-old self. By combining my medical records for accuracy with that of my personal perception of my journey, I wanted to reflect both sides of what I was faced with at the time and my less rational, instant thoughts in response to the facts I was presented with. I felt that writing about my hospital admission and Olivia's funeral using a poetry format would allow the intensity of my emotions to unravel at the same pace as those scenes unfolded, as well as it enabling me to better describe how they felt to endure.

When I look back to the start of my stillbirth journey now, I realise the underlying desperation behind my personal need to put the pieces of what happened together, at the same time as trying to ensure that everybody around me could carry on as "normal" without having to worry about me. Although this makes me feel somewhat saddened, I feel that my personal account gives an insight that is very true to that time and exposes the grief and emotions that I went through personally.

Throughout the course of the years that have followed my stillbirth, my journey has taken me through a couple of crossroads, but has guided me through many new and exciting chapters. I recently read a blog about pregnancy following a loss, so I feel it is imperative to give a glimpse into my own experience of this:

> "During the months that followed Olivia's death, I found myself constantly reminded of my loss. Although I made the decision to go back to work to avoid a prolonged maternity leave without my little girl, I felt lost as my heart and arms continued to physically ache for my baby. Each time I switched on the television or left the house I couldn't help but notice pregnant women and newborn babies. The few clothes and blankets I had bought for Olivia whilst I was pregnant, not only served as a reminder of the part of my life that I had lost, but gave me the clarification of the part of my life that I still yearned for. Facing a heightened chance of developing pre-eclampsia and HELLP syndrome

during a future pregnancy was daunting, but when I met with a consultant in the August to discuss both what I had just been through and the risks involved with any future pregnancies, I was already pregnant. During the appointment, I found out that I had a blood clotting disorder called 'Prothrombin Gene Mutation', which is an inherited condition. We inherit one copy of each blood clotting gene from our parents and, in my case, one of my genes was faulty. This means that during times where there is generally an increased chance of developing a blood clot; such as pregnancy, after surgery and after long flights, my chances of developing a blood clot are higher. I was given medical compression socks to wear throughout my pregnancy and was told that I would have to inject myself with a blood thinner for six weeks after my baby was born. I left the appointment with the comfort that although my pregnancy was high risk, it would be consultant-led.

From the time of Olivia's funeral and into the start of my following pregnancy, I had a recurring anxiety around death and experienced vivid dreams of being buried alive. As my pregnancy progressed, I felt the same happiness and excitement I had felt whilst pregnant with Olivia. In many ways there was no difference between either of my pregnancies as I still enjoyed following my baby's development and mulled over baby names. In some ways, though, my excitement was tainted with a heightened worry as I knew all too well how quickly my last pregnancy had changed. I also felt an underlying guilt, which at times could be quite conflicting. I felt guilty having another baby so soon after Olivia had died. I didn't want anybody to forget about her and I definitely wasn't replacing her, but if I spent too much time at the cemetery or felt too conscious of the thought that I was betraying Olivia, I would then start to feel guilty towards the baby I was carrying as I didn't want him or her growing up in Olivia's shadow as such. The confliction in my mind continued throughout my pregnancy. When I got to fourteen weeks I fainted. Although I was worried, at the same time it was something different about this pregnancy which gave me hope in some ways, yet terrified me in others.

The milestones of my new pregnancy were bittersweet too. The reassurance of hearing my baby's heartbeat and feeling the movements of my growing baby also reminded me of going through the same milestones with Olivia and highlighted such a fine line between life and death.

At twenty weeks, I found out that I was having a little boy, and from this point onwards I had a lot of extra appointments and ultrasounds at the hospital. The consultant that led my pregnancy was always very reassuring and I remained well cared for by the staff at the hospital. I felt like a ticking time bomb, wondering if I was going to die and, although I hoped more than anything that I would have my baby at the end of my pregnancy, I also didn't dare to think about it too much. As I passed the point in my pregnancy that I had lost Olivia, I felt a combination of relief as the days and weeks elapsed, but felt vulnerable going through these previously unknown stages of pregnancy.

I made it to thirty-seven weeks and thought it would be the right time to buy the larger items that I had held back on, such as a pram, just in case I did get to bring my baby home. However, whilst I was out, I suffered a placental abruption due to an undetected blood clot behind the placenta. Although this brought back many fears initially, as yet again my pregnancy had taken a sudden and unexpected turn with a similar twist of being taken by ambulance to the nearest hospital, once I had heard my baby's heartbeat and had that knowledge that he was alive, I felt hopeful and could see the outcome that I hadn't dared think about in sight.

My labour progressed quickly this time. Although I did experience this complication at the very end of my pregnancy, my little boy, Oliver, was born safely and I had got through my pregnancy pre-eclampsia and HELLP syndrome free!"

Despite finding myself juggling conflicting guilt between Olivia and Oliver initially, I quickly came to realise that it is okay to be a mother to both of my children. I feel continuously blessed to share my life with Oliver, and for the opportunities that he gives me to learn and to grow.

This year marked the eighth anniversary since I lost Olivia, and I am still as much her mum as I was at the time of her stillbirth. I continue to be thankful for my time with Olivia, which allows me to fulfil my role as her mother in many different and positive ways. In Olivia's memory, I have done fundraisers and set up a JustGiving page to raise funds for the unit at the hospital that cared for us. This currently stands at £2,609.37. I am also a registered volunteer at the same hospital. I have signed up as a blood donor and given blood, trained in first aid from birth up to adulthood and designed a webpage around stillbirth and Christmas time, which I hope to work on with an appropriate charity. I continue to help at an annual baby memorial service, which again I hope to expand on; I am also trying to change body labels in current use for babies after my experience with Olivia and hope to work with a pre-eclampsia charity in the future.

The years seem to have flown by and I have learned a lot from my experiences. As I look to the future, I hope that the work I continue to do as Olivia's mother can make a difference to other families. In regards to stillbirth, I hope that something positive can be taken from my experiences and that the taboo surrounding stillbirth can become that much more lifted. I would like to conclude by sharing the following poems that I have written around the emotions of stillbirth, but also say that by allowing that acknowledgement to somebody either going through or remembering the loss of their baby, instead of brushing it under the carpet, may just be the light that is needed to shine through even the darkest of days.

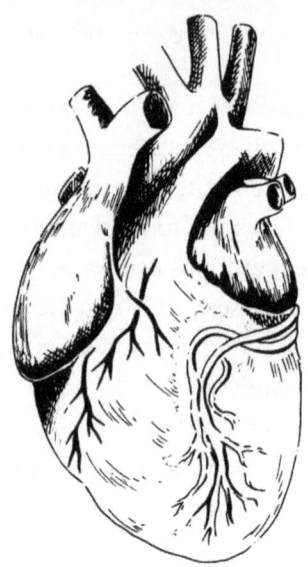

Battle of the Heart

There's a pain in my heart, at the centre of my chest,
It constantly feels like a cardiac arrest,
The protective sac not doing its job,
Shattering my heart with every throb,
Pressure builds up as my veins start to close,
No design in the chambers designed for my woes,
Backflow prevented, valves stubborn and mean,
Rhythm is disturbed, but circulation is keen,
Arteries declare exit guiding the blood,
A state of emergency, "Heart bleeding more than it should"!
An undercover operation that no-one can see,
Unknown to the world not a way to set free,
Still standing its ground beating, to keep me alive,
Mission complete though it's tough, my heart battles to survive.

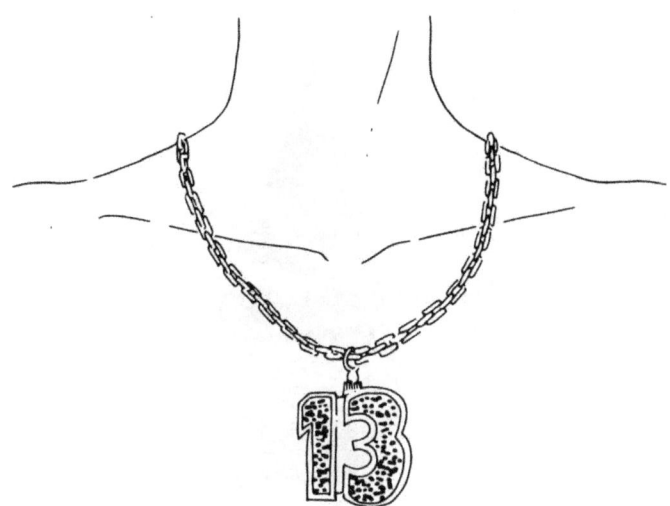

Number Thirteen

Bad luck and misfortune are places I've been,
Around my neck it seemed hung the number thirteen,
But through all of the bad, the good has shined through,
An invisible ring on my finger, still commits me to you.

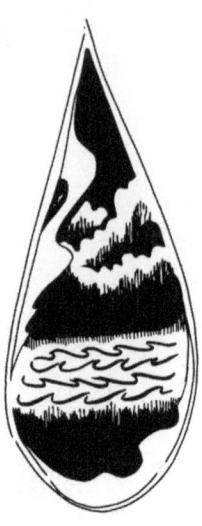

The Journey of a Teardrop

As soon as the teardrop fell from my eye,
It travelled on a journey, lost under the sky,
Holding my sadness, my misery and pain,
Taking my story to fall with the rain,
If only it knew it can't bring you back,
Magical it is, but superpowers are lack,
Determined it continues its way to the sea,
Battling all odds, still fighting for me,
Reaching the ocean, it's tiny but strong,
The sun catches a glisten, though its journey was long,
So next time the sea sparkles, don't wonder why,
It's made up of teardrops, with their stories they lie.

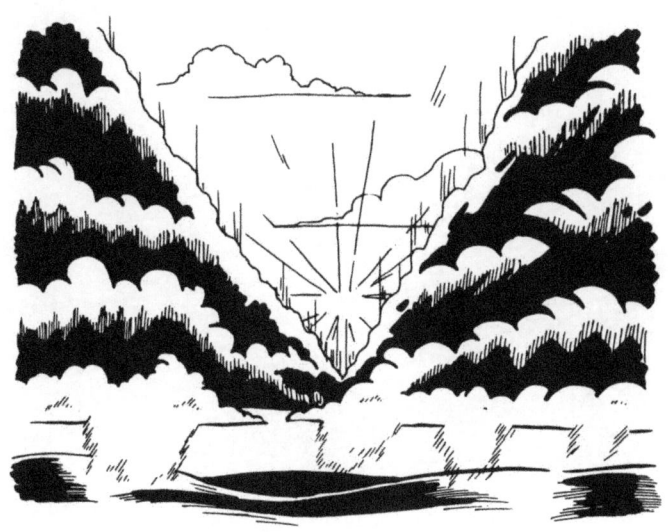

Rainbow of Hope

Somewhere amongst the dull, heavy clouds.
Where the sky is grey and still.
There's a rainbow.
Putting colour into the gloom.
Creating beauty as it stretches through the misery of the open sky.
So when it seems that the world is surrounded by dark,
And when unhappy clouds not only cry but weep to the ground below.
Search for that rainbow.
And when you find the alluring colours that creep through the uncertainty.
With it you will find hope.

References

Cummings, J., and Bennett, V. (2012) *Compassion in Practice: Nursing, Midwifery and Care Staff – Our Vision and Strategy.* NHS Commissioning Board, Leeds. http://tinyurl.com/c5lc4n2 (accessed 26th March 2014).

Downe, S., Schmidt, E., Kingdon, C., Heazeall, A.E.P. (2013) *Bereaved Parents' Experience of Stillbirth in UK Hospitals: a qualitative interview study,* BMJ Open. 2013; 3(2): e002237. Published online 2013 Feb 14. doi: 10.1136/bmjopen-2012-002237 PMCID: PMC3586079

Redshaw, M., Rowe, R. & Henderson, J. (2014) *Listening to Parents after Stillbirth or the Death of their Baby.* National Perinatal Epidemiology Unit, London: University of Oxford.

NHS Choices https://www.nhs.uk/conditions/pre-eclampsia/causes/

Tommy's https://www.tommys.org/pregnancy-information/pregnancy-complications/pre-eclampsia-information-and-support

Action on Pre-Eclampsia https://action-on-pre-eclampsia.org.uk/public-area/pre-eclampsia-information/hellp/#1464715167988-138a3f3f-0e3e

NICE Guidelines https://pathways.nice.org.uk/pathways/hypertension-in-pregnancy#path=view%3A/pathways/hypertension-in-pregnancy/pre-eclampsia.xml&content=view-index https://www.nice.org.uk/Search?q=Pre-eclampsia

SANDS https://www.sands.org.uk/about-sands/who-we-are/why-sands-exists

Melbourne haematology http://www.melbournehaematology.com.au/fact-sheets/prothrombin-gene-mutation.html

Acknowledgements

I would like to express my gratitude to the following people who have travelled alongside me throughout the journey of writing this book and beyond:

Firstly to all at Troubador Publishing who have advised, listened and guided me thoroughly through the publication process. I couldn't have entrusted a better team. Thank you especially to Hannah Dakin for all of your support and advice, Rosie Lowe for orchestrating the production process from manuscript to book, Alexa Davies for all of your invaluable marketing work and input and Andrea Johnson for your work and distribution of the eBook version.

Nik, for all of your hard work designing and producing the book cover and to all at Book Beaver who contributed to the illustrations. For being enthusiastic, approachable, hardworking and above all professional, thank you.

Chris Navin, for encouraging me to write a book and for writing the foreword! Thank you for your continued support in all that I do and for believing in me throughout the course of the years. There are so many unsung heroes within the NHS and you are one of them.

Oliver, my hero, my world and my best friend. Thank you for enriching my life. You give me courage and strength and inspire me to do better each day, I love you.

Grandma, thank you for being there for me. I will never forget the time that you came to see Olivia and you gave me the silver heart pendant to give to her, which I placed over her heart. Your words at the time touched me and meant a lot.

Katherine, for your continued support and belief in me throughout the years. I couldn't have wished for a better friend, thank you.

Mum and Dad, thank you for being there for me. Sophie and Charlotte, always believe in the journey ahead and take knowledge from what can be learned.

Samantha and David, thank you for taking the time to read through my manuscript.

Jan Owen, for the privilege of being able to work alongside you over the years and for your friendship. Thank you.

Mandy and Geoff, thank you for your guidance.

Thank you to Kate Davie's at Tommy's charity for taking the time to talk through the pre-eclampsia and HELLP syndrome sections and for providing me with helpful, friendly and professional advice.

And finally, to each and every person who has supported my fundraising campaign and to every reader of this book. Thank you.